FROM MANAGING TO CONQUERING BLOATHING

Expert Guide To Understanding Causes, Symptoms, and Tailored Treatment Plan For Optimal Wellness

DR. DASHIELL DANIEL

Disclaimer

This book, is intended to provide information and guidance on the subject matter and is not a substitute for professional medical advice, diagnosis, or treatment.

The author does not own or endorse any such entities mentioned in the book. Any resemblance to actual persons, living or dead, or actual events is purely coincidental.

Readers are encouraged to consult with qualified healthcare professionals for medical advice, diagnosis, and treatment tailored to their specific circumstances.

The author and the publisher disclaim any liability for any loss or risk, personal or otherwise, arising directly or indirectly from the use of the information presented in this book.

By reading this book, the reader acknowledges and agrees to the terms of this disclaimer.

"BLOATING" is a book that tackles a widespread and frequently disregarded health issue that impacts people from different backgrounds.

This thorough handbook proves to be an invaluable tool for comprehending, treating, and avoiding bloating in the modern world of increased health awareness. This book is significant because it carefully examines all the facets of bloating, from its definition and typical symptoms to the complex digestive processes that are involved.

By dissecting the varieties of bloating, explaining their numerous components, and exploring the intricacies of the digestive system, Chapter 1 lays the groundwork for the rest of the book. Information is presented in a way that not only improves reader understanding but also makes it easier to understand the complex material methodically.

The common causes of bloating are examined in Chapter 2, where they are divided into three categories: nutritional, lifestyle, and medical. Through analyzing the complex interactions between factors such as dietary fibers, fructooligosaccharides, and stress, the book offers a sophisticated comprehension that is essential for efficient handling.

The importance of the text becomes even more apparent in Chapter 3, which covers the diagnostic terrain of bloating. It provides information about medical testing as well as self-assessment techniques, enabling readers to take an active role in their health. The focus on using self-evaluation to identify trigger foods is in line with current developments in customized health.

The value of the book is increased by Chapters 4 and 5, which discuss management and prevention techniques and the situations in which professional assistance is necessary, respectively. For readers looking for practical answers, the integration of food tactics, lifestyle modifications, and medicinal interventions offers a comprehensive approach.

In Chapter 6, the complex relationship between bloating and mental health is explored from a novel angle. The story gains depth when the gut-brain connection is acknowledged and coping mechanisms for psychological issues are provided, recognizing the holistic nature of health.

Lastly, Chapter 7's practical components—such as hydration advice and dishes that are bloating-friendly—transform theoretical knowledge into doable actions. Meal plans and recipes are included, which not only improves the information's accessibility but also makes the book more useful as a daily guide.

"BLOATING" provides thorough, well-researched, and approachable guidance to a common health condition, therefore surpassing the traditional bounds of health literature. It is an essential resource for readers in general and healthcare professionals in particular, as it empowers people to actively participate in their well-being in addition to spreading knowledge.

First Of All

Bloating is a frequent physiological phenomenon that is often uncomfortable. It is defined as an abnormal distention or swelling of the belly brought on by the buildup of gas or fluid. This illness is common in a variety of populations and can be brought on by several things, from underlying medical issues to dietary choices. It is important to comprehend bloating for people who are trying to alleviate its symptoms as well as for medical professionals who are trying to identify and treat related conditions. In this in-depth investigation, we tackle the complex features of bloating, including its definition, importance, and wide-ranging topic.

What Bloating Means

Examining the condition's complexity is necessary to define bloating. Bloating is commonly identified by an apparent distention and a subjective sensation of fullness, tightness, or swelling in the abdomen. The accumulation of gas, liquid, or a combination of the two in the digestive tract is the main cause of this feeling. From a physiological perspective, bloating may result from problems with gas control, changes in the gastrointestinal tract's motility, or heightened sensitivity to appropriate gas concentrations. Bloating must be distinguished from other gastrointestinal symptoms, such as discomfort or pain in the abdomen, as these may have distinct underlying causes and therapeutic consequences.

Understanding Bloating Is Important

Because bloating affects so many people and negatively affects their quality of life, it is crucial to comprehend. People all across the world, regardless of age, gender, or location, complain about bloating. Bloating discomfort can cause several detrimental effects, such as decreased productivity at work, a decline in social involvement, and difficulties in day-to-day functioning. Furthermore, underlying gastrointestinal conditions such as small intestinal bacterial overgrowth (SIBO), irritable bowel syndrome (IBS), and inflammatory bowel disease (IBD) may be indicated by persistent bloating.

By deciphering the complexities of bloating, medical practitioners can improve patient outcomes by sharpening their diagnostic skills and customizing interventions to target the underlying causes.

The Book's Scope

This book is not just about bloating as a symptom; it's also a comprehensive investigation of its relationships to a range of physiological and psychological issues. The book explores the various causes of bloating, such as gut microbiota function, gastrointestinal motility issues, and food triggers. It also examines the psychological components of bloating, recognizing the reciprocal relationship between gastrointestinal symptoms and mental health. The difficulties in diagnosing bloating are also examined, emphasizing the need to distinguish between organic and functional reasons. A thorough discussion of therapeutic approaches is included, encompassing everything from medication to lifestyle changes, offering a thorough manual for medical professionals and anyone suffering from bloating. This book seeks to provide readers with a more sophisticated understanding of the complex interactions that lead to bloating, going beyond traditional viewpoints and ultimately enabling better management and results for those who experience this common gastrointestinal ailment.

CHAPTER ONE
UNDERSTANDING BLOATING

Bloating is a frequent gastrointestinal symptom that is defined by an abdomen-wide feeling of fullness, tightness, or distension. It is a personal experience with variable duration and intensity that has an impact on people for various reasons. Abnormal gas buildup in the digestive tract is one of the main reasons for bloating. This gas can be produced by several processes, including the digestion of undigested food by colonic bacteria, which releases gases like hydrogen and methane. Bloating and water retention in the abdominal tissues can also be linked, which makes the abdomen feel heavy and uncomfortable. To effectively manage and alleviate this common digestive problem, it is imperative to investigate the varied causes of bloating and understand the underlying mechanisms causing it.

Bloating is the term used to describe the subjective feeling of fullness and tightness in the abdomen, which is frequently accompanied by visual distension. This phenomenon is a complicated and multidimensional symptom that can arise for several reasons. Bloating is frequently caused by excessive gas buildup, water retention, and specific food allergies. The fermentation of undigested carbohydrates in the colon can result in gas buildup and the formation of gases such as hydrogen, carbon dioxide, and methane. In contrast, water retention refers to the abnormal build-up of fluid in the abdominal tissues, which results in a discernible increase in circumference. Furthermore, bloating may result from dietary allergies as the body reacts to specific substances, causing gastrointestinal tract discomfort and inflammation.

Bloating can have a wide range of causes, all of which have an impact on the digestive system. One common cause of abdominal distension is the fermentation of carbohydrates by bacteria in the colon, which results in the breakdown of undigested food and the production of gasses. Moreover, poor nutrition absorption and digestion might result in the buildup of compounds that ferment in the stomach, causing bloating to worsen. Bloating can also be caused by elements including a sedentary lifestyle, drinking too little water, and having specific medical conditions.

It is crucial to comprehend the complex interactions between these elements to develop focused management and prevention methods for bloating.

Bloating is commonly related to a variety of discomforts that people may have daily. The classic symptoms of bloating include visible abdominal distention, increased gas, and abdominal pain or cramping. Additionally, people may express sensations of fullness, tightness, and overall discomfort in the abdomen. Individual differences in severity might be seen in the intermittent or chronic nature of these symptoms. Accurate diagnosis and the development of customized interventions to address the unique causes of bloating in each case depend on the ability to recognize and comprehend these symptoms.

There are various ways that bloating can present itself, and each has its traits and causes.

A frequent form of bloating called "water retention" is caused by an abnormal build-up of fluid in the tissues, which makes the swelling and pain noticeable. This type of bloating is frequently linked to changes in hormone levels, kidney disease, or other illnesses that impair fluid balance.

Another common kind of bloating is gas buildup, which is caused by bacteria in the colon fermenting undigested carbs. Gases produced by this process have the potential to distension and discomfort in the abdomen. Furthermore, bloating associated with food sensitivities is a result of an unpleasant reaction to particular dietary ingredients, which in vulnerable individuals causes inflammation and bloating.

One form of bloating that is strongly related to the body's fluid balance management is water retention.

The body's capacity to maintain an ideal fluid balance can be impacted by several factors, including sodium intake, renal function, and hormonal variations. An imbalance of this kind can cause extra fluid to build up in the tissues of the abdomen, which can cause bloating and discomfort. Hormonal fluctuations, especially during the menstrual cycle, can cause women to retain water in their bodies, which can lead to weight swings and distension in the abdomen.

To address this particular form of bloating and carry out focused therapies to restore fluid balance, it is imperative to comprehend the mechanisms underlying water retention.

Bloating which is commonly associated with gas accumulation is typified by the accumulation of gases within the digestive tract. The colon's bacterial fermentation of undigested carbohydrates is the cause of this occurrence.

The gases that are produced—carbon dioxide, methane, and hydrogen—contribute to pain and distension in the abdomen. The degree of gas accumulation can be influenced by variables like food choices, intestinal transit speed, and the makeup of the gut microbiota. Gas-related bloating may be more noticeable in people with diseases like small intestinal bacterial overgrowth (SIBO) or irritable bowel syndrome (IBS). For efficient management and relief from the symptoms of bloating, it is imperative to address the underlying causes of gas accumulation.

Food sensitivities are a major factor in the appearance of bloating and can cause discomfort in the digestive system in those who are vulnerable. Bloating and inflammation are caused by unfavorable reactions that some foods might cause in the gastrointestinal tract. Frequently identified as contributing factors are lactose, gluten, and certain kinds of carbohydrates that are not well absorbed in the small intestine.

For instance, the incapacity of those who are lactose intolerant to digest lactose might cause bloating and the generation of gas. Similar to this, bloating may be a symptom of a gluten-sensitive person's body's immunological reaction to gluten-containing foods. The key to controlling bloating brought on by food allergies and enhancing overall digestive health is recognizing and avoiding trigger foods.

Comprehending the mechanisms behind bloating requires an understanding of the digestive process. Digestion is a multifaceted physiological process that breaks down food into nutrients that may be absorbed. Food is first broken down mechanically and enzymatically in the mouth before passing into the stomach and small intestine to be further broken down and nutrients absorbed. Undigested food travels to the gut microbiota in the colon, where bacteria ferment carbohydrates and release gasses.

Bloating can be caused by disturbances in the digestive process at any point, underscoring the significance of a comprehensive strategy for maintaining digestive health.

Many factors that affect how well nutrients are broken down and absorbed can affect the complex process of digestion. Digestion can be impacted by dietary decisions, meal composition, and the rate at which the stomach empties.

For instance, inadequate chewing may prevent food from being mechanically broken down in the mouth, which could cause bigger particles to enter the stomach and small intestine. Additionally, the effective breakdown of proteins, lipids, and carbohydrates depends on the availability of specific digestive enzymes. Any imbalances or shortages in these enzymes have the potential to impair digestion and exacerbate bloating. Identifying probable causes of bloating and developing focused therapies require a thorough understanding of the factors controlling digestion.

A complex ecology of bacteria living in the gastrointestinal tract, the gut microbiome is essential to both general health and digestive function. Bloating may result from the fermentation of undigested carbohydrates in the colon, which is facilitated by the microbiome and produces gasses.

Antibiotic usage, along with lifestyle and dietary choices, all have an impact on the variety and makeup of the gut microbiome. Dysbiosis, or imbalances in the microbiome, can upset the delicate environment and cause bloating and stomach problems. Beneficial bacteria called probiotics can support a balanced microbial environment, which in turn can help manage bloating and contribute to a healthy gut microbiome. Investigating the complex interaction between bloating and the gut flora offers important insights into prospective treatments for enhancing digestive health.

In summary, bloating is a complex symptom that can be caused by several variables, such as increased gas production, water retention, and dietary sensitivity. It is essential to comprehend the many sorts and reasons for bloating to effectively manage and alleviate this widespread digestive discomfort. The process of digestion,

CHAPTER TWO
COMMON CAUSES OF BLOATING

One common gastrointestinal symptom is bloating, which can be caused by a variety of causes including nutrition, lifestyle, and underlying medical issues. Knowing the many causes is important for those who are looking for relief as well as for medical experts who want to treat this widespread issue.

Dietary issues are a major contributing cause of bloating. Foods high in fiber, which are frequently praised for their advantages to the digestive system, might, ironically, make some people feel bloated. Some fibers are fermentable, which can produce gas during digestion and cause distension in the abdomen. Furthermore, bloating may be brought on by consuming fermentable oligosaccharides, disaccharides, monosaccharides, and polyols (FODMAPs), particularly in those who are sensitive. Known for their fizz, carbonated drinks cause the digestive tract to absorb carbon dioxide, which increases gas and causes bloating. Artificial sweeteners, which are frequently used to replace sugar, can also cause stomach disturbances and bloating in those who are vulnerable.

Another important aspect that contributes significantly to bloating is a lifestyle.

The accumulation of gas in the gastrointestinal tract can be caused by a sedentary lifestyle, which is defined as a lack of physical exercise. Underappreciated in their effects on physical well-being, stress, and worry can disrupt digestive processes and cause bloating in certain people. The gut-brain axis, a complex relationship between the brain and the stomach, emphasizes how crucial mental wellness is to digestive health. Moreover, sleep deprivation, a widespread problem in modern culture, can interfere with digestive processes and make bloating sensations worse.

One intricate aspect of the etiology of bloating is medical problems. The symptoms of Irritable Bowel Syndrome (IBS), a functional gastrointestinal illness, include bloating, changed bowel habits, and abdominal pain. Since the precise mechanisms causing IBS are yet unknown, managing the condition can be difficult. Abdominal pain and bloating are among the symptoms of Inflammatory Bowel Disease (IBD), which includes diseases such as Crohn's disease and ulcerative colitis. IBD is characterized by a persistent inflammation of the digestive tract. Bloating is a common symptom of Celiac Disease, an autoimmune condition brought on by gluten ingestion. Bloating is a symptom of underlying intestinal illnesses, which can be brought on by bacteria, viruses, or parasites that interfere with normal digestion processes.

In summary, bloating is a complex symptom with a variety of underlying causes. Abdominal distension may result from dietary decisions involving the ingestion of high-fiber meals, FODMAPs, carbonated beverages, and artificial sweeteners. Bloating is primarily caused by lifestyle factors that interfere with digestion processes, such as stress, lack of sleep, and a sedentary lifestyle.

The intricacy of the etiology of bloating is further highlighted by underlying medical diseases such as gastrointestinal infections, Celiac disease, inflammatory bowel disease, and irritable bowel syndrome. For bloating to be effectively managed and relieved—whether by dietary changes, lifestyle alterations, or focused medical interventions—a thorough understanding of these many aspects is necessary.

CHAPTER THREE
BLOATING DIAGNOSIS

The procedure of diagnosing bloating is complex and entails both medical testing and self-evaluation. Bloated people frequently self-evaluate as a first step in determining possible triggers and patterns related to their symptoms.

Self-Evaluation

Maintaining a Food journal: Keeping a thorough food journal is a frequently used technique for self-evaluation. This entails keeping a thorough record of all the food types, portion quantities, and meal times that are consumed each day. People who keep a diet journal can see links between certain foods and the beginning of bloating. By taking a thorough approach, it is possible to uncover dietary trends that may be linked to bloating and make educated changes to eating habits.

Finding Trigger meals: One of the most important parts of self-evaluation is figuring out which meals can make bloating symptoms worse. Bloating can result from eating certain foods, such as those high in fermentable carbs, which promote gas production.

People can try cutting back on or removing particular food groups to see how that affects their bloating. This method of self-observation gives people the ability to make knowledgeable food decisions, which helps to create a customized strategy for controlling and preventing bloating.

Medical Examinations

Medical tests are an important diagnostic tool for bloating in addition to self-assessment since they offer a more thorough and objective examination of the underlying causes.

Breath tests for Small Intestinal Bacterial Overgrowth (SIBO): An increased number of bacteria in the small intestine that is not normal is the hallmark of SIBO, a medical disorder.

The hydrogen breath test is one of the breath tests that is frequently used to diagnose SIBO.

People drink a certain substrate during this test and the analysis of breath gasses that follows aids in the identification of bacterial overgrowth. With the use of this diagnostic test, medical personnel can identify SIBO as a possible source of bloating and utilize that information to guide specific interventions for bacterial imbalance.

Endoscopy and colonoscopy: These are useful diagnostic techniques that provide a more direct view of the gastrointestinal tract.

During an endoscopy, the stomach, upper portion of the small intestine, and esophagus are examined by passing a flexible tube equipped with a camera through the mouth or nose.

A colonoscopy examines the colon and rectum while concentrating on the lower gastrointestinal tract. By using these techniques, medical professionals can find anomalies that could be causing bloating, such as tumors, ulcers, or inflammation.

Tailored treatment strategies are made possible by the accurate diagnosis obtained from endoscopic examinations.

Blood testing: Blood testing is crucial for assessing different signs that could point to underlying health issues that are causing bloating. Increased inflammatory marker levels, including C-reactive protein, may indicate gastrointestinal tract inflammation. Additionally useful in ruling out additional possible causes such as infections or autoimmune illnesses are blood tests. Healthcare providers can identify a patient's underlying health issues and guide additional investigations by using blood parameter analysis to help differentiate between bloating and other conditions.

In summary, a mix of medical testing and self-evaluation is used to diagnose bloating. Self-assessment techniques, such as maintaining a food journal and identifying trigger foods, enable people to spot trends and make wise dietary decisions. Medical practitioners can discover underlying causes such as SIBO, gastrointestinal problems, or inflammatory disorders with objective data from breath tests, endoscopy, and blood testing. This all-encompassing method guarantees an extensive assessment, facilitating a more precise diagnosis and the creation of focused treatment plans for bloating patients.

CHAPTER FOUR
MANAGING AND BLOATING PREVENTION

Bloating is a prevalent gastrointestinal ailment that is distinguished by an abdominal area sensation of fullness and tightness, frequently accompanied by apparent distension. Bloating can have a variety of causes, from dietary modifications to underlying medical disorders. An all-encompassing strategy that includes dietary modifications, lifestyle adjustments, and, in certain situations, prescription drugs or medical procedures is needed to manage and prevent bloating.

Dietary tactics are essential for controlling bloating, and the Low-FODMAP (Fermentable Oligosaccharides, Disaccharides, Monosaccharides, and Polyols) diet is one such strategy that works well. This diet plan calls for limiting the consumption of specific carbohydrates that are fermented by bacteria in the colon and poorly absorbed in the small intestine, causing bloating and gas production. This diet restricts foods that are high in lactose, fructose, and certain fibers. According to research, following a low-FODMAP diet can help people with irritable bowel syndrome

(IBS) and other functional gastrointestinal disorders dramatically reduce their symptoms of bloating.

Consuming live beneficial bacteria through the use of probiotics is another dietary approach that can have a good impact on gut flora. An imbalance in the gut microbiota can lead to bloating.

The gut microbiota is essential for digestion and the fermentation of certain chemicals. Probiotics may be able to assist in bringing this balance back, which would lessen gas production and ease the symptoms of bloating. However individual reactions and the effectiveness of particular probiotic strains can differ.

Supplementing with enzymes is another dietary strategy to control bloating.

Enzymes included in these supplements help break down proteins, lipids, and carbs to make digestion easier.

Enzyme supplements may lessen gas production and bloating by improving digestion and lowering the possibility that undigested food will enter the colon and ferment. These supplements may be helpful for people who have shortages in particular digestive enzymes or illnesses that impair the activity of enzymes.

Apart from food tactics, alterations in lifestyle can also have a substantial effect on bloating. Frequent physical activity and exercise encourage regular bowel movements and lower the risk of constipation, which is a common cause of bloating. The gastrointestinal tract's muscles are stimulated by exercise, which helps food and waste pass through the digestive system. Aerobic exercise, like jogging or walking, can be very helpful for decreasing bloating and enhancing digestive health.

Since stress can worsen gastrointestinal symptoms, stress management strategies are essential for treating bloating. Prolonged stress can change the sensitivity, secretion, and motility of the gut, which can aggravate bloating and other digestive problems.

Stress-reduction methods including yoga, meditation, and deep breathing have been demonstrated to lessen bloating symptoms. Those who are prone to stress-related bloating may find it especially helpful to incorporate stress management into everyday routines.

Another crucial lifestyle component that affects digestive health and bloating is getting enough sleep. Reduced vulnerability to gastrointestinal disturbances and changes in the makeup of the gut microbiota has been linked to poor sleep quality and inadequate sleep duration.

In addition to potentially lowering bloating, maintaining a regular sleep schedule, practicing good sleep hygiene, and making sure you get enough sleep are all factors in overall digestive health.

Medication and other medical interventions may be taken into consideration in situations where food and lifestyle changes are insufficient. Medication available over the counter, like simethicone, relieves bloating by dissolving gas bubbles in the digestive system. These drugs are usually well tolerated and are frequently used to treat symptoms. However, different people may respond differently to them.

If underlying issues are the cause of your bloating, your doctor may give prescription drugs such as prokinetics and some that target your gut hormones. Prokinetics increases the motility of the gastrointestinal tract, which lessens the chance of food fermentation and stagnation.

Drugs that affect gut hormones can affect different parts of the digestive system and may help relieve the symptoms of bloating that are related to certain illnesses.

When using prescription drugs, one must carefully evaluate their health situation as well as any possible adverse effects.

Surgical treatments may be investigated in cases of severe and persistent bloating that are unresponsive to other interventions.

Bloating-causing structural anomalies in the gastrointestinal tract can be addressed with procedures like laparoscopic surgery. Nevertheless, surgical treatments are usually limited to certain medical conditions, and the choice to proceed with surgery is decided after a comprehensive evaluation of the patient's health and symptoms and in conjunction with medical professionals.

treating and avoiding bloating requires a comprehensive strategy that takes into account dietary tactics, lifestyle modifications, and, if required, prescription drugs or other medical procedures. Optimizing results requires adjusting interventions to the unique preferences of each patient as well as the underlying reasons for bloating. For those who have this common gastrointestinal ailment, an integrative strategy that incorporates dietary changes, lifestyle adjustments, and, when necessary, medical advice can greatly improve the overall management of bloating and improve quality of life.

CHAPTER FIVE
APPLICATIONS OF PROFESSIONAL HELP

Bloating is a typical gastrointestinal symptom that is defined by a feeling of fullness, constriction, or edema in the abdomen. Periodic bloating is usually not harmful and might be related to food choices or transient digestive problems, but if symptoms are severe or chronic, medical assistance may be necessary.

Understanding warning signs and when to consult a medical professional are essential for early identification and successful treatment of underlying bloating disorders.

An important warning indication for bloating is persistent symptoms. Bloating that occurs sometimes after eating a certain food may be common, but if it continues for a long time, there may be underlying health problems. Irritable bowel syndrome (IBS), inflammatory bowel disease (IBD), and other gastrointestinal illnesses may be the cause of persistent bloating. When bloating becomes chronic and negatively affects everyday functioning and quality of life, seeking professional assistance becomes essential.

Another warning sign that people who are experiencing bloating should be aware of is unexplained weight loss. Even though bloating by itself could not cause weight loss, persistent bloating combined with inexplicable weight loss may indicate a more serious underlying illness, such as malabsorption problems or gastrointestinal cancers. Fast and inadvertent weight loss necessitates a medical assessment every once to determine and treat the underlying reason.

The presence of blood in the stool is a serious indicator of bloating. Visible blood in the stool, known as hematochezia or melena, may be a sign of gastrointestinal bleeding. Bleeding can result from conditions including gastrointestinal ulcers, inflammatory bowel disease, or colon cancer, and when bloating and blood in the stool occur together, medical assistance must be sought right once. Finding and treating the underlying cause of gastrointestinal bleeding requires prompt action.

For an accurate diagnosis and successful treatment, selecting the appropriate healthcare provider is crucial when considering obtaining professional assistance for bloating. As the initial point of contact for bloated people, primary care physicians (PCPs) are vital. PCPs are qualified to provide baseline assessments, request pertinent testing, and offer first advice.

A referral to a gastroenterologist can be required if the cause of the bloating is still unknown or calls for specific knowledge. As experts in digestive system issues, gastroenterologists can do more thorough examinations, including endoscopies and imaging tests, to determine the underlying cause of bloating and its accompanying symptoms.

When it comes to treating bloating, registered dietitians can be invaluable members of the healthcare team. Bloating is frequently caused by dietary issues; a qualified dietitian may evaluate a person's diet, pinpoint possible triggers, and suggest individualized dietary changes.

Dietary assessments can identify conditions like lactose intolerance, celiac disease, or specific food intolerances, and making the right dietary adjustments can greatly reduce the symptoms of bloating.

knowing when to seek medical attention for bloating is critical. Red flags include persistent symptoms, unexplained weight loss, and blood in the stool. Primary care physicians serve as the first point of contact, offering advice and initial assessments. For more complicated situations, gastroenterologists provide specialist knowledge and undertake thorough investigations to determine the underlying cause of bloating.

To reduce bloating, registered dietitians evaluate dietary components and provide customized dietary recommendations. Effective bloating management and the resolution of any potential underlying health issues depend on prompt and appropriate contact with healthcare providers.

CHAPTER SIX
BLOATING AND MENTAL HEALTH

There is a complex and nuanced interaction involving both physiological and psychological factors between bloating and mental health. Investigating the relationship between the stomach and the brain reveals that digestive processes can be greatly impacted by mental health. Stress is a typical occurrence in modern life and has been shown to have a strong impact on digestion. Emotional and psychological moods can affect gastrointestinal functioning because of the two-way communication allowed by the complex network of neurons and biochemicals that make up the gut-brain axis. The body triggers the "fight or flight" response during stressful situations, directing resources away from digestion and toward urgent survival requirements. This rerouting may result in worse digestion and exacerbate bloating symptoms.

One important part of the gut-brain relationship is how stress affects digestion. Stress hormones like cortisol are released when the sympathetic nervous system is activated. Changes in gut motility, greater visceral sensitivity, and modifications to the gut microbiota have all been linked to elevated cortisol levels. All of these elements work together to cause bloating and other gastrointestinal complaints.

Chronic stress can also worsen intestinal inflammation, which further impairs the digestive tract's ability to function. Recognizing the connection between digestive and mental health, managing bloating can be approached more comprehensively when the impact of stress is understood.

Mind-body methods become useful resources for reducing stress-related bloating. Techniques including progressive muscle relaxation, deep breathing, and mindfulness meditation have shown promise in regulating the stress response. In particular, mindfulness promotes people to develop a judgment-free awareness of the present moment, which can offset the physiological consequences of stress on digestion by fostering a sense of calm. By incorporating these approaches into everyday routines, bloating symptoms can be lessened and overall mental health can be improved, strengthening the interaction between the mind and the gut.

The emotional components of bloating that either cause or follow from bloating episodes are explored in the psychological elements of bloating. Anxiety is a common mental health issue that is closely related to gastrointestinal symptoms, such as bloating. Once again, the gut-brain axis is crucial because elevated anxiety can lead to aberrant gut contractions, heightened sensitivity to distension, and changes in the makeup of the gut flora. Bloating can be made worse by maladaptive coping mechanisms that people with anxiety may display, such as changing their eating habits or avoiding particular foods.

Holistic management requires coping mechanisms for the bloating brought on by anxiety. It has been established that cognitive-behavioral therapy (CBT) is a successful treatment strategy for treating bloating associated with anxiety.

To help people manage their anxiety and how it affects their gastrointestinal symptoms, cognitive behavioral therapy (CBT) tries to recognize and alter maladaptive thought patterns and behaviors. Furthermore, people can exercise conscious control over physiological processes by using relaxation techniques like guided imagery and biofeedback, which fosters a sense of agency in controlling bloating. Incorporating these psychological therapies into treatment programs promotes overall well-being by acknowledging the bidirectional nature of the gut-brain link.

the complex relationship between bloating and mental health emphasizes the significance of approaching its comprehension and treatment from a holistic perspective. Because of the dynamic interaction established by the gut-brain connection, digestive processes can be influenced by stress and anxiety, which may exacerbate sensations of bloating. Mind-body methods and psychological therapies are useful ways to lessen the influence of mental health issues on bloating, highlighting the relationship between mental and physical health. Identifying and treating the psychological as well as the physiological aspects of bloating is essential to creating comprehensive and successful plans that support mental health in general and digestive health in particular.

CHAPTER SEVEN
RECIPES FOR BLEACHING RELIEF

By making thoughtful food choices, bloating—a prevalent and frequently irritating gastrointestinal symptom—can be lessened. Creating meal plans that are specifically designed to reduce bloating is a complex process that takes into account different elements of digestion and nutrient absorption. When it comes to bloating-friendly meal plans, it's critical to pay attention to how breakfast, lunch, and dinner are prepared and to include appropriate snack alternatives. Easy-to-digest foods including lean proteins, whole grains, and low-FODMAP (fermentable oligosaccharides, disaccharides, monosaccharides, and polyols) alternatives should be the focus of these diets. Creating customized meal plans that effectively relieve bloating requires taking into account each person's unique dietary preferences and sensitivities.

Friendly Meal Plans For Bloating

When creating meal plans to reduce bloating, it is important to consider the particulars of each meal. Breakfast might be as simple as low-fat yogurt with berries, porridge with sliced banana, or a smoothie made with easily digested fruits and greens. Adding grilled chicken with quinoa and steamed vegetables, salmon with sweet potatoes, or a stir-fried vegetable dish with tofu to your lunch or dinner will help you avoid bloating while still getting the nutrients you need. Rice cakes with nut butter, cucumber slices with hummus, or a small portion of low-FODMAP fruit are a few possible snack options. The secret to effective bloating reduction is to tailor meal plans to each person's preferences and tolerances.

Fluid Requirements And Bloating

Drinking enough water is essential for maintaining digestive health and can have a big effect on bloating. Selecting the correct drinks is essential to promoting healthy digestion and lowering the risk of bloating episodes. Teas made from herbs, which are well known for their calming effects, can help reduce bloating. For example, peppermint tea has long been used to aid easier digestion and relieve gastrointestinal discomfort. Tea made with chamomile, which has anti-inflammatory qualities, is another great option. Moreover, thinking about infused water recipes improves hydration and provides the body with vital nutrients. Adding cucumber, mint, and lemon to water not only gives it a delicious twist, but it also contains components that help reduce bloating. You may promote intestinal well-being by including these water measures in your everyday routine.

Herbal Teas

One particularly useful ally in the fight against bloating is herbal tea. Made from the leaves of the Mentha piperita plant, peppermint tea has menthol, a muscle relaxant that can lessen bloating and alleviate intestinal spasms.

The dried flowers of the Matricaria chamomilla plant are used to make chamomile tea, which is well known for its anti-inflammatory properties that soothe the digestive system and reduce bloating discomfort. The rhizome of the Zingiber officinale plant is used to make ginger tea, which is prized for its capacity to promote digestion, lessen gas, and ease bloating. Including these herbal drinks in everyday activities will help prevent bloating symptoms before they arise.

Recipes For Infused Water

There's more to being hydrated than just drinking plain water; try these tasty and health-boosting infused water recipes. For example, water infused with cucumber, mint, and lemon has all the pleasant qualities of lemon and mint combined with the moisturizing qualities of water. Because of its high water content, cucumber helps you stay hydrated, while mint helps your digestive system feel better. Because of its alkalizing qualities, lemon may aid in bringing the pH levels in the stomach into balance. This infusion delivers a blast of natural flavors and digestive benefits in addition to encouraging higher water intake. By experimenting with different infused water recipes, people may customize how hydrated they are while also taking care of their bloating issues.

In summary, treating bloating necessitates a multifaceted strategy that goes beyond simple dietary changes. Creating meal plans that are conducive to bloating requires careful evaluation of foods, with an emphasis on selections that are easily digested and avoiding known triggers. Drinking herbal teas and ingeniously blended water concoctions helps you stay hydrated, which is very beneficial for your digestive system. Customizing these tactics to meet each person's tastes and tolerances guarantees a successful and individualized method of relieving bloating. Through the integration of these ideas into everyday routines, people can effectively mitigate and reduce the discomfort that comes with bloating, thus promoting enhanced digestive health and general well-being.

CONCLUSION

An improper buildup of gas in the digestive tract causes bloating, a complicated physiological phenomenon that causes discomfort and a bloated abdomen. Numerous factors, such as dietary practices, gastrointestinal issues, and lifestyle decisions, might contribute to this illness.

It's important to comprehend the fundamental ideas around bloating for both patients looking for relief and medical experts trying to treat its underlying causes.

Digestive Physiology: Gas is a normal result of this intricate biochemical process that breaks down food into absorbable nutrients during the digestive process. When there is a disruption in the regular digestion and absorption of nutrients, bloating may result. Gas buildup can be caused by several factors, including poor digestion of some carbohydrates, changed gut flora, and reduced motility of the digestive tract. Understanding the causes underlying bloating and creating focused therapies require a solid understanding of gut physiology.

Dietary Influences: Food is a major factor in bloating, and some food items can either make symptoms worse or better. A class of carbohydrates known as fermentable oligosaccharides, disaccharides, monosaccharides, and polyols (FODMAPs) are poorly absorbed in the small intestine and have the potential to ferment in the colon, producing gas. Furthermore, by altering transit time and bacterial fermentation, meals heavy in fat and fiber might aggravate bloating. Effective bloating management requires analyzing individual food patterns and providing tailored suggestions based on nutritional science.

Gastrointestinal illnesses: A wide range of gastrointestinal illnesses, from more serious ailments like inflammatory bowel disease (IBD) to functional disorders like irritable bowel syndrome (IBS), can be linked to bloating. Specifically, IBS is frequently characterized by bloating, altered bowel patterns, and discomfort in the abdomen. Accurate diagnosis and focused treatment plans depend on an understanding of the pathophysiology of these illnesses, which includes the roles played by immune system regulation, visceral hypersensitivity, and gut-brain connections.

Microbiota and Dysbiosis: The intricate community of bacteria that live in the digestive system, known as the gut microbiota, is essential to preserving gut health. Dysbiosis, or changes in the variety and composition of the microbiota, has been connected to several gastrointestinal symptoms, including bloating. Stress, food, and antibiotic use are a few examples of factors that might affect the equilibrium of gut flora. Investigating the complex link between bloating and the microbiota offers insights into prospective treatment strategies, like probiotics and prebiotics.

Psychosocial Factors: The interaction between the central nervous system and the gut's enteric nervous system is emphasized by the gut-brain axis. Bloating and other gastrointestinal symptoms can be greatly impacted by stress, anxiety, and other psychological factors that affect gastrointestinal function. For a complete approach to reducing bloating, it is imperative to comprehend the interplay between the mind and the gut. Stress-reduction methods and cognitive-behavioral therapies could be beneficial elements of a multimodal treatment program.

Diagnostic Difficulties: Because bloating is complex and its symptoms often overlap with those of other gastrointestinal disorders, diagnosing it can be difficult. It takes a methodical and thorough approach, including a thorough clinical history, physical examination, and diagnostic testing, to accurately identify the underlying causes. Difficulties in distinguishing between organic and functional reasons highlight the significance of using modern diagnostic techniques in conjunction with clinical judgment to provide a precise diagnosis.

Treatment Plans: Each person's unique contributing variables must be addressed in a customized plan for managing bloating. Pharmacological therapy, nutritional interventions, and lifestyle adjustments are frequently utilized. Successful management requires identifying and treating the underlying causes, which may include food triggers or gastrointestinal issues.

Treatment plans that are comprehensive and patient-centered are guaranteed when healthcare specialists from several professions collaborate on patient care.

Patient education and empowerment: Encouraging people to take an active role in their care requires educating them about bloating, its causes, and the various available management techniques. Making educated decisions about food choices, lifestyle adjustments, and possible triggers is made easier when clear and reliable information is provided.

Furthermore, encouraging candid communication between patients and healthcare professionals promotes a team-based strategy for bloating management, improving treatment compliance and overall results.

In summary, bloating is a complex phenomenon that is influenced by a wide range of variables, such as microbiota, psychosocial variables, gastrointestinal illnesses, dietary habits, and diagnostic difficulties. To properly diagnose and treat bloating, healthcare providers must have a thorough awareness of these ideas.

Through individualized and interdisciplinary methods, healthcare providers can improve the quality of life for patients experiencing bloating and promote overall gastrointestinal health and well-being by treating the underlying reasons.

www.ingramcontent.com/pod-product-compliance
Lightning Source LLC
Chambersburg PA
CBHW071124260726
48661CB00006B/2690